SIRTFOOD DIET

COOKBOOK

FOR BEGINNERS

A COMPLETE GUIDE FOR BEGINNERS TO LOSE WEIGHT FAST, BURN FAT, GET LEAN, BOOST METABOLISM WITH EASY-TO-MAKE AND HEALTHY RECIPES
{7-DAY MEAL PLAN, 21-DAY MEAL PLAN AND COOKBOOK}

LENORA SAWYER

Copyright

Table of Contents

Introduction

You can lose weight, and you can do so in a way that is safe and healthy and without leaving out all the foods you might enjoy. There are many diets to choose from, but the sirtfood diet is one that at the moment is getting plenty of attention. This diet focuses on sirtuins-proteins that will help you achieve the results you were looking for with yourself. Celebrities have praised this diet. Singer Adele has recently reported to have lost almost 100 pounds. Using the green juice that we will mention, along with exercise, on the sirtfood diet. You can activate fat loss ad help in preventing yourself from suffering from all kinds of diseases by using sirtfood-rich foods in your diet and enjoying them regularly.

You will use sirtuins on the sirtfood diet - those proteins that will help your body control its metabolism. Some plant-based foods are considered to be filled with sirtuins, and are therefore assumed to be the secret to rapidly losing weight. Strawberries, dark chocolate, green tea, and even red wine are filled with these higher levels of sirtuins that you can enjoy to make you feel good while consuming nutritious foods that will keep your energy levels boosted. And, certain foods that are rich in sirtuins are also delicious.

Although, there are alternatives that can help you lose weight, why not take advantage of a way your body functions naturally? You can start losing weight quickly and easily by eating those sirtuin-rich foods, or "sirtfoods," significantly when you exercise and restrict calories. As a result, you'll be able to lose weight, and with the sirtfood diet, people have been found to lose weight while still retaining the same muscle mass they had before, which means they remain healthy and strong, regardless of weight loss. Typically, there is a change in muscle mass during weight loss that can be very troublesome for those who are attempting to retain their strength.

If you want to follow this diet or move on to another diet it is up to you at the end. This diet is, of course, very strict, particularly in the first week, but it does ease up, and during the day you can find yourself able to enjoy many different meals and snacks, some recipes will be given that are intended to keep you as safe as possible while still producing the results you are searching for.

What is the sirtfood diet?

Nutritionists Aiden Goggins and Glen Matten founded the Sirtfood Diet. They were so interested in the potential of Sirtfoods that they developed a diet focused on optimizing the intake of Sirtfood and mild restriction of calories. They then tried this diet on participants from an elite gym in London and were shocked by their results. In the first 7 days, gym participants lost an average of 7 pounds, despite not increasing their rate of exercise. The participants lost a huge amount of weight and developed muscle (usually the reverse occurs while dieting) and showed substantial changes in overall health and well-being.

What are Sirtuins?

Sirtuins are proteins within your cells that are there to regulate them. Typically, they are tasked with being able to maintain cellular homeostasis. This means that their jobs are to make sure that your cells stay exactly how they should be. They are meant to make sure that your body is consistent and that your cells' consistency can be easily maintained. Because your body is designed to work within very specific parameters that are maintained during homeostasis, you need something to keep those parameters set. Just as homeostasis keeps your temperature just right to avoid allowing bacteria to run rampant in your body as well as your brain cooking if your body got too hot, sirtuins work within your body to make sure that you are kept within the right constant as well. The result is that you get a sort of cellular homeostasis.

On the sirtfood diet, you fast and restrict calories. This tells your body to change how to respond to food. The sirtuins tell your body to respond differently. Instead of working to uptake the energy and store it as fat, your body is told to reject the fats, along with the cholesterol as well. As a result, your body burns the fats and cholesterol through oxidation. That allows the fat to be used up, burned, and then lost. This works to then allow you to lose the weight that you were trying to cut.

However, because sirtuins want to keep things the same, they can then tell the body to continue functioning as normal. Through doing so, you end up seeing that the body continues to function at those higher levels. You see that the body is actually going to actively burn calories instead of clinging to them in the form of fat. The sirtuins will allow for the body to continue burning off that fat, and as a result, you continue to lose weight despite the severe degree of caloric restriction.

So how does the sirtfood diet work?

The diet is divided into 2 stages. First Phase: the 'hyper success phase' of 7 days, which involves a Sirtfood-rich diet with mild calorie reduction, and Second Phase: the 'maintenance phase' of 14 days, in which you consolidate your weight loss without limiting calories.

The First phase of the sirtfood diet

The calorie intake is limited to 1,000 calories for the first 3 days. There are 3 Sirtfood-rich green juices and 1 Sirtfood-rich meal and 2 dark chocolate squares in the diet.

The calorie intake is raised to 1, 500 calories for the remaining 4 days and 2 Sirtfood-rich green juices and 2 Sirtfood-rich meals are included in the diet per day.

You cannot drink any alcohol during Phase 1, but you are free to drink water, tea, coffee, and green tea.

The second phase of the sirtfood diet

The second phase does not rely on limiting calories. Three Sirtfood-rich meals and 1 green juice are included each day, plus the option of 1 or 2 irtfood bite snacks if desired.

You are permitted to drink red wine in phase 2, but in moderation (2-3 glasses of red wine per week are recommended), as well as water, tea, coffee and green tea.

What are the sirtfoods?

Mostly plant-based and rich in antioxidants, Sirtfoods help trick the body at a higher rate to burn fat. It is called Sirt because it involves consuming foods that are rich in activators of sirtuin, defined as seven proteins that control metabolism, inflammation, and cell longevity found in the body.

The top 20 sirtfoods as: arugula, buckwheat, capers, celery, chilies, chocolate, coffee, extra virgin olive oil, garlic, green tea, kale, Medjool dates, parsley, red endive, red onion, red wine, soy, strawberries, turmeric and walnuts.

What happens after you have completed the sirtfood diet?

Sirtfood Diet isn't planned as a one off 'diet', but rather a way of living. If you have completed the first 3 weeks, you must continue consuming a Sirtfood-rich diet and continue drinking your daily green juice. It is suggested that the first and second phases can be repeated for a health boost if and when needed, or if things have gone a little off track.

Are there any side effects to the sirtfood diet?

It can cause exhaustion, nausea, diminished mental concentration, and headaches if you're not used to eating so little during the day. This diet can also lead to bad breath, which can result from not eating enough.

What else should you eat?

Sirtfoods should be supplemented with protein. Stop overloading processed and sugary foods, as well as mercury-high fish.

These are also recommended foods, in addition to the sirtfoods: vegetables, fruits, nuts, grains, beans, herbs and tea in one's diet. Asparagus, bok choy, green beans, blackberries, goji berries, kumquats, raspberries, chia seeds, peanuts, popcorn, quinoa, cinnamon and ginger

Side effects to the Sirtfood Diet?

If you're not opened to eating little during the day, it can cause fatigue, nausea, impaired mental focus & headaches, says Smith.

This diet may also lead to some unpleasant bowel movements if you're not eating enough fibe, you might get bad breath.

Healthy Sirtfood Diet Recipes are below;

Enjoy, lose weight and stay healthy!

Yields: 15 to 20 Servings

Recipes:

- ¼-cup of cocoa nibs or 1 ounce dark chocolate (85percent cocoa solids) also broken into pieces

- One teaspoon vanilla extract or Scraped seeds of one vanilla pod

- One cup of walnuts

- One tablespoon of cocoa powder

- One tablespoon of extra-virgin olive oil

- Nine-ounces Medjool dates (pitted)

- One to two tablespoons of water

- One tablespoon of ground turmeric

Directions

1. In a food processor put the walnuts and chocolate, Afterwards; process it until you have a fine powder.

2. Add all other recipes except water and mix until ball is well mixed. Considering the consistency of the mixture you may or may not have to apply water (you wouldn't want it to be too sticky).

3. Shape the mixture into bite-size balls with your hands and then refrigerate in an airtight container for one hour at least before eating them.

4. You may roll some of the balls to a particular finish in a little more cocoa or dried cocoa. They can hold in your fridge for up to one week.

Sirt Super Salad

Yields: 1 Serving

Recipes:

- Three and a half ounces of smoked salmon slices

- 1 3/4 ounces of arugula

- Half cup celery including leaves (sliced)

- ¼ cup of parsley (chopped)

- 1 ¾ ounces of endive leaves

- One tablespoon of capers

- Half cup avocado (peeled, stoned & sliced)

- One large Medjool date (pitted and chopped)

- ⅛ cups of walnuts (chopped)

- One tablespoon of extra-virgin olive oil

- ¼ lemon juice

- ⅛ cups of red onion (sliced)

Directions

1. Place the salad leaves on a clean bowl or in a big clean container.

2. Mix all the left recipes together and top of the with leaves.

Miso-Marinated Baked Cod with Stir-Fried Greens & Sesame

Yields: 1 Serving

Recipes:

- One tablespoon of mirin

- Three and a half teaspoons of miso

- 1 by 7-ounce skinless cod fillet

- 1/8 cup of red onion (sliced)

- 3/8 cup of celery (sliced)

- One tablespoon of extra-virgin olive oil

- Two garlic cloves (finely chopped)

- One Thai chili (finely chopped)

- One teaspoon of fresh ginger (finely chopped)

- 3/8 cup of green beans

- 1/4 cup of buckwheat

- One teaspoon of sesame seeds

- Two tablespoons of parsley (roughly chopped)

- One teaspoons of ground turmeric

- One tablespoon of tamari (or soy sauce, for gluten-free)

- 3/4 cup of kale (roughly chopped)

Directions:

1. Preheat the oven to 425 degrees Fahrenheit. Mix the mirin, one teaspoon of the oil and miso. Rub all the cod and leave for about 30 mins to marinate.

2. After you've done that, bake the cod for approximately 10 mins.

3. Heat up a big frying pan or wok with the rest of the oil. You should then add the onion and stir-fry for some mins, then add the garlic, kale, chili, green beans, ginger, and celery. Toss and fry until the kale becomes tender and well cooked through. You will

have to add some water to the pan to support the process of cooking.

4. Cook the buckwheat together with the turmeric (according to package directions).

5. Add the parsley, tamari and sesame seeds to the stir-fry and then serve with fish and buckwheat.

Aromatic Chicken Breast with Kale, Red Onions and A Tomato & Chili Salsa

Yields: 1 Serving

Recipes:

- Two teaspoons of ground turmeric

- ¼ lemon juice

- One teaspoon of fresh ginger (chopped)

- One tablespoon of extra-virgin olive oil

- ⅛ cup of red onion (sliced)

- ⅓ cup of buckwheat

- ¼-pound of chicken breast (skinless & boneless)

- ¾ cup of kale (chopped)

For The Salsa:

- 1⁄4 lemon juice

- One Thai chili (finely chopped)

- One tablespoon capers (finely chopped)

- One medium tomato

- Two tablespoons parsley (finely chopped)

Directions

1. To prepare the salsa, remove the eye from the tomato and slice it very finely, ensuring the liquid stays as large as possible. Mix the capers, chili, lemon juice and parsley together. You can put it all in a clean blender, but the final outcome might be a little different.

2. Preheat the oven to 425 degrees Fahrenheit. In one teaspoon of turmeric, the lemon juice and a little oil,

marinate the chicken breast. Leave for about five to ten minutes.

3. Heat the ovenproof frying pan till heat is high, then add the marinated chicken to each side for a minute, until it appears pale golden, then move to the oven (ensure to place on a baking tray if it is not ovenproof) for eight to ten minutes, or until well cooked. Take out from the oven, gently cover with foil, and leave for five minutes before serving it.

4. In the meantime, in a steamer cook kale for about five minutes. Fry the ginger and the red onions in some little oil, until it becomes soft but also not browned, and then add the cooked kale and fry for some additional minute.

5. Cook the buckwheat with the remaining turmeric teaspoon according to product directions. Serve together with the vegetables, salsa and chicken.

Asian Shrimp Stir-Fry with Buckwheat Noodles

Yields: 1 Serving

Recipes:

- Two teaspoons of tamari (or soy sauce, for gluten-free)

- Half cup of chicken stock

- Two teaspoons of extra-virgin olive oil

- Half cup of green beans (chopped)

- Two garlic cloves (finely chopped)

- One Thai chili (finely chopped)

- Three-ounces of soba (buckwheat noodles)

- 1/8 cup of red onions (sliced)

- 1/3-pound of shelled raw jumbo shrimp (deveined)

- One teaspoon of fresh ginger (finely chopped)

- 3/4 cup of kale (roughly chopped)

- Half cup of celery including leaves (trimmed & sliced, with leaves put separately)

Directions

1. Heat up a large clean frying pan over high heat, in one teaspoon of the oil and one teaspoon of the tamari, cook the shrimp for about two to three minutes.

2. You should then transfer the shrimp to a dish. Using a paper towel carefully wipe out the pan. You'll use again.

3. In boiling water cook the noodles for five to eight minutes or as instructed on the package. Remove water and then put aside.

4. Afterwards, fry the chili, red onion, ginger, celery (don't include leaves), kale, green beans and garlic in the rest of the tamari and oil over medium to high

heat for approximately two to three mins. Having done that, add the stock and then bring to a boil also simmer for one to two mins, until the vegetables are cooked but remain crunchy.

5. Add the noodles, celery leaves and the shrimp to the pan, then bring back to a boil, then take away from the heat and then serve.

Strawberry Buckwheat Tabbouleh

Yields: 1 Serving

Recipes:

- Half cup of avocado

- One tablespoon of extra-virgin olive oil

- 3⁄4 cup of parsley

- 1⁄8 cup of red onion

- 1⁄8 cup of Medjool dates (pitted)

- One tablespoon of ground turmeric

- One tablespoon of capers

- 3⁄8 cup of tomato

- 1⁄3 cup of buckwheat

- Half lemon juice

- 2⁄3 cup of strawberries (hulled)

- One-ounce arugula

Directions

1. Cook the buckwheat with the remaining turmeric teaspoon according to product directions. Remove water and then put aside to let cool.

2. Afterwards, finely chop the tomato, parsley, dates, capers, red onion and avocado and then mix with the cooked buckwheat.

3. Also slice the strawberries and carefully mix into the salad with the lemon juice and oil. Serve on a bed of arugula to enjoy.

Sirtfood Green Juice

Yields: 1 Serving

Recipes:

- One big handful arugula
- Half level teaspoon matcha powder
- Two to Three large celery stalks (including leaves)
- One very small handful flat-leaf parsley
- Two big handfuls kale
- Half to One-inch piece of fresh ginger
- Half lemon juice
- Half medium green apple

Directions

1. Mix the parsley, kale and arugula together, juice them well enough afterwards before moving to other ingredients. The aim is to get about 2 fluid ounces or close to 1/4 cup of the juice.

2. At this time juice the apple, ginger and celery.

3. Peel the lemon and maybe put it through the juicer although it is easier to just squeeze gently the lemon by hand into the juice. At this phase, you should have about one cup of juice or just a little more.

4. You add the matcha when the juice is ready to be served. In a glass pour a little quantity of juice, and then add the matcha, stir strongly using a teaspoon or fork.

5. As soon as the matcha gets dissolved, add the rest of the juice. Stir one more time, and then enjoy the drink. Top with plain water or just as you desire.

Turmeric Chicken & Kale Salad with Honey Lime Dressing

Yields: 2 Servings Overall Time: 30 mins

Recipes:

For the Chicken:

- Nine-ounces chicken mince or diced up chicken thighs

- One large garlic clove (finely diced)

- Half teaspoon of salt plus pepper

- One teaspoon of turmeric powder

- Half medium brown onion (diced)

- One teaspoon of ghee or one tablespoon of coconut oil

- Half lime juice

- One teaspoon of lime zest

For the salad:

- One handful of fresh parsley leaves (chopped)

- Three large kale leaves (stems removed & chopped)

- Half avocado (sliced)

- Six broccolini stalks or Two cups of broccoli florets

- Two tablespoons pumpkin seeds (pepitas)

- One handful of fresh coriander leaves, chopped

For the dressing:

- One small garlic clove, finely diced or grated

- Three tablespoons of lime juice

- One teaspoon of raw honey

- Half teaspoon of sea salt plus pepper

- Half teaspoon of wholegrain or Dijon mustard

- Three tablespoons of extra-virgin olive oil

Directions

1. Heat up or coconut oil or the ghee in a clean small frying pan over medium to high heat. Add the onion and then sauté on medium heat for four to five minutes, until it appears golden. Add the garlic and chicken mince and then stir for two to three mins over medium to high heat, breaking it away from each other.

2. Add the lime zest, turmeric, pepper, salt and lime juice and then cook, frequently stirring, for an additional three to four mins. Put aside the cooked mince.

3. As the chicken is cooking, bring a clean small saucepan of water to boil. Add the broccolini and then cook for two mins. Afterwards, rinse under cold water and also cut into about three to four pieces each.

4. Add the pumpkin seeds carefully to the frying pan from the chicken and then toast over medium heat for 2 mins, frequently stirring to avoid burning. Season with some salt. Put away. You can use raw pumpkin seeds too.

5. Place the chopped kale in a clean salad bowl and then pour over the dressing. Toss and massage the kale using your hands with the dressing. It will soften the kale.

6. Lastly toss through the broccolini, fresh herbs, cooked chicken, avocado slices and pumpkin seeds.

Notes:

To prepare fast, dress the salad ten mins before serving. Bee mince can be used in place of Chicken, fish or chopped prawns. Cooked quinoa or chopped mushrooms can be used by vegetarians.

Buckwheat Noodles with Chicken Kale & Miso

Yields: 2 Servings Overall Time: 30 mins

Recipes:

For the noodles:

- Five-ounces buckwheat noodles (no wheat)

- Two to Three handfuls of kale leaves (stem removed & roughly cut)

- One long red chilli, thinly sliced (seeds in or as desired)

- One teaspoon of coconut oil or ghee

- One brown onion (finely diced)

- One medium free-range chicken breast (sliced or diced)

- Two to Three tablespoons Tamari sauce (or soy sauce, for gluten-free)

- Three to Four shiitake mushrooms (sliced)

- Two large garlic cloves (finely diced)

For the miso dressing:

- One tablespoon of Tamari sauce

- One teaspoon of sesame oil (if desired)

- One and a half tablespoon fresh organic miso

- One tablespoon of lemon or lime juice

- One tablespoon of extra-virgin olive oil

Directions

1. Bring a clean medium saucepan of water to boil. Add the kale and cook for one min, until it is slightly wilted. Remove and put aside but reserve the water andthen bring it back to the boil. Add the soba noodles and then cook according to the package directions (usually abt five mins). Rinse under cold water and set aside.

2. In the meantime, carefully pan fry the shiitake mushrooms in coconut oil (abt one teaspoon) or a little ghee for two to three minutes, until lightly browned on all side. Sprinkle with some sea salt and then put aside.

3. In the same frying pan, heat more ghee or coconut oil over medium to high heat. Sauté chilli and onion for two to three mins and add the chicken pieces afterwards. Cook for five mins over medium heat, stirring a couple of times, then add the tamari sauce, garlic and some water. Cook for an additional two to three mins, frequently stirring until chicken is well cooked.

4. Lastly, add the soba noodles and kale and then toss through the chicken to heat up.

5. Now mix together the miso dressing and drizzle over the noodles right at the end of cooking and serve to enjoy.

Asian King Prawn Stir-Fry With Buckwheat

Yields: 1 Serving

Recipes:

- Two teaspoons of tamari (or soy sauce for gluten-free)

- 75grams of soba (buckwheat noodles)

- One garlic clove (finely chopped)

- 50grams of kale (roughly chopped)

- One bird's eye chilli (finely chopped)

- One teaspoon of fresh ginger (finely chopped)

- Two teaspoons of extra virgin olive oil

- 150grams of shelled raw king prawns (deveined)

- 20grams red onions (sliced)

- 40grams celery (trimmed & sliced)

- 5grams of lovage or celery leaves

- 75grams green beans (chopped)

- 100ml chicken stock

Directions

1. Heat up a clean frying pan over a high heat, and then cook the prawns in one teaspoon of the oil and one teaspoon of the tamari for two to three mins. The prawns should be transferred to a plate afterwards. Using a paper towel wipe out the pan, it'll be used again.

2. Proceed to cook the noodles in boiling water for five to eight minutes or according to package directions. Remove water and put aside.

3. In the meantime, fry the chilli, garlic, ginger, beans and celery, kale and red onion in the rest of the oil over medium to high heat for two to three mins. Afterwards, Add the stock and bring to the

boil, then simmer for one or two minutes, until the vegetables are well cooked but sremains crunchy.

4. Add the noodles, lovage or celery leaves and prawns to the pan, bring back to the boil and then remove from the heat. Serve to enjoy.

Baked Salmon Salad With Creamy Mint Dressing

Yields: 1 Serving Overall Time: 20 mins

Recipes:

- One salmon fillet

- 40grams of mixed salad leaves

- 40grams of young spinach leaves

- Two radishes (trimmed & thinly sliced)

- 50g of cucumber (cut into chunks)

- Two spring onions (trimmed & sliced)

- One small handful of parsley (roughly chopped)

For the dressing:

- One teaspoon of low-fat mayonnaise

- One tablespoon of natural yogurt

- One tablespoon of rice vinegar

- Two leaves mint (finely chopped)

- Salt

- Freshly ground black pepper

Directions

1. Firstly you should heat up the oven to 200
   degrees Celsius.

2. Place the salmon fillet on a clean baking tray and
   then bake for about sixteen to eighteen mins. The
   salmon goes well in the salad either hot or cold.
   Salmon with skin will require you cook with skin
   side down. A fish slice can be used to remove the
   salmon skin after cooking. It should slide off
   easily when cooked.

3. In a clean small container, mix together the
   yogurt, rice wine vinegar, mint leaves, salt,
   pepper and mayonnaise together and let it stand

for a minimum of five minutes to allow the

flavors get deeper.

4. Place the spinach and salad leaves on a dishing

    plate and then top with the cucumber, parsley,

    spring onions and radishes. Gently flake the

    cooked salmon onto the salad and then drizzle

    the dressing over to enjoy.

Choc Chip Granola

Yields: 8 Servings Overall Time: 30 mins

Recipes:

- 50grams of pecans (roughly chopped)

- 200grams of jumbo oats

- 60grams dark chocolate chips

- Three tablespoons of light olive oil

- One tablespoon of dark brown sugar

- 20grams of butter

- Two tablespoons of rice malt syrup

Directions:

1. Heat up the oven to 160 degrees Fahrenheit. Line a clean large baking tray with a silicone sheet or baking parchment.

2. Mix the pecans and oats together in a clean big container. In a clean small non-stick pan, gently heat the butter, olive oil, rice malt syrup and brown sugar until the butter is melted and the syrup and sugar have also dissolved. Ensure not to allow it boil. Afterwards, pour the syrup over the oats and vigorously stir until the oats are fully covered.

3. Arrange the granola over the baking tray, arranging in the corners. Now leave clumps of mixture with spacing rather than an uniform spread. Bake in the oven for twenty mins until it appears tinged golden brown at the edges. Take out from the oven and then leave on tray to let cool completely.

4. When it gets cool, using your fingers, ensure there aren't any bigger lumps on the tray and

having done that mix in the chocolate chips.

Scoop the granola into an airtight jar. You can

store granola for a minimum of two weeks.

Fragrant Asian Hotpot

Yields: 2 Servings Overall Time: 15 Mins

Recipes:

- 1/4 teaspoon of ground anise or One star anise (crushed)

- One teaspoon of tomato purée

- A small handful of coriander (10grams, stalks finely chopped

- 50grams cooked water chestnuts (drained)

- Half of lime juice

- 100grams firm tofu, (chopped)

- One tablespoon of good-quality miso paste

- 500ml chicken stock (either fresh or made with one cube)

- Half carrot (peeled & cut into matchsticks)

- 50grams broccoli (cut into small florets)

- A small handful of parsley (10grams, stalks finely chopped)

- 50grams beansprouts

- 20grams sushi ginger (chopped)

- 100grams raw tiger prawns

- 50grams rice noodles (cooked according to direction on pack)

Directions

1. Place the star anise, tomato purée, coriander stalks, parsley stalks, chicken stock and lime juice in a clean big pan and then bring to a simmer for about ten mins.

2. Add the broccoli, carrot, tofu, noodles, water chestnuts and prawns and gently simmer until the prawns are well cooked. Take away from the heat and then stir in the miso paste and sushi ginger.

3. You should serve sprinkled with the coriander

leaves and parsley.

Lamb,Butternut Squash And Date Tagine

Yields: 4 Servings Overall Time:1 hour 30 mins

Recipes:

- One red onion (sliced)

- Two tablespoons of olive oil

- Three garlic cloves (either grated or crushed)

- 400grams tin chopped tomatoes, plus half a can of water

- One teaspoon of chilli flakes (or as desired)

- Two tablespoons of fresh coriander (plus extra for garnish)

- 2-cm ginger (grated)

- 500grams butternut squash (chopped into 1-cm cubes)

- Two teaspoons of cumin seeds

- One cinnamon stick

- Two teaspoons of ground turmeric

- 800grams lamb neck fillet (cut into chunks about 2-cm)

- Buckwheat, couscous, flatbreads or rice (Serving purpose)

- 100grams medjool dates (pitted & chopped)

- 400grams tin chickpeas (drained)

- Half teaspoon of salt

Directions

1. Heat up the oven to 140 degrees C.

2. In a clean large ovenproof saucepan or cast iron casserole dish drizzle about two tablespoons of olive oil. Afterwards, add the sliced onion, with the lid on cook on a gentle heat for approximately five

minutes, until the onions becomes soften but isn't brown.

3. Add the ginger and grated garlic, cumin, chilli, turmeric and cinnamon. Stir and then cook for additional one minute with the lid off. If it gets too dry you can add a splash of water.

4. Add in the lamb chunks. Stir slowly to coat the meat in the spices and onions, afterwards, add the chopped dates, tomatoes and salt, and also about half a can of water.

5. Bring the tagine to the boil, having done that, put the lid on and place in the heated oven for 1 hr 15 mins.

6. When it is about 30 minutes to the end of the cooking time, add in the drained chickpeas and chopped butternut squash. Stir all, put the lid back

on and then return to the oven for the last time, About 30 mins.

7. When the tagine is set, take out of the oven and then stir through the chopped coriander. You should serve with couscous, buckwheat, basmati rice or flatbreads.

Notes

You can simply cook the tagine in a clean saucepan or cast iron casserole dish if you don't have an ovenproof saucepan, until it is needed to go inside the oven & gently transfer the tagine into a regular clean lidded casserole dish before placing in the oven. With an additional 5 mins cooking time to allow for the fact that the casserole dish will require additional time to heat up.

Prawn Arrabbiata

Yields: 1 Serving Overall Time: 1 hr 15 mins

Recipes:

- 125grams raw or cooked prawns

- 65grams Buckwheat pasta

- One tablespoon of extra virgin olive oil

For Arrabbiata Sauce:

- One Garlic clove (finely chopped)

- 40grams Red onion (finely chopped)

- 30grams Celery (finely chopped)

- One Bird's eye chilli (finely chopped)

- One teaspoon of Extra virgin olive oil

- 400grams Tinned chopped tomatoes

- One teaspoon of Dried mixed herbs

- One tablespoon of Chopped parsley

* Two tablespoon of White wine (if desired)

Directions

1. Fry the garlic, onion, chili, celery and also the dried herbs in the oil over a medium to low heat for one to two minutes. Increase the heat up to medium, and then add the wine and cook for one minute. Having done that, add the tomatoes and then leave the sauce to simmer over a medium to low heat for twenty to thirty minutes, until it has a lovely consistency. You can some water if the sauce is too thick.

2. Just as the sauce is cooking bring a pan of water to the boil and then cook the pasta following to the packet directions. After you've cooked it as desired, drain, toss with the olive oil and then leave in the pan until it will be required.

3. If using raw prawns, add them to the sauce and cook

    for a further three to four mins, until they have

    turned pink and also opaque, add the parsley and

    then serve. If using cooked prawns add them with

    the parsley, bring the sauce to the boil and serve.

4. Add the pasta (cooketo the sauce, mix but carefully

    and then serve.

Turmeric Baked Salmon

Yields: 1 Serving Overall Time: 30 Mins

Recipes:

- One teaspoon of Extra virgin olive oil

- 150grams of Skinned Salmon

- 1/4 lemon Juice

- One teaspoon of ground turmeric

For the spicy celery:

- 40grams of Red onion (finely chopped)

- One teaspoon of Extra virgin olive oil

- 1-cm of ginger (fresh & finely chopped)

- One Bird's eye chili (finely chopped)

- 150grams Celery (cut into 2-cm lengths)

- One Garlic clove (finely chopped)

- One teaspoon of mild curry powder

- 130grams of Tomato (cut into eight wedges)

- 60grams of Tinned green lentils

- One tablespoon of Chopped parsley

- 100ml Chicken or vegetable stock

Directions

1. Preheat the oven to 200 degrees Celsius.

For the spicy celery:

1. Heat up a clean frying pan over a medium to low heat, add the olive oil, then the onion, garlic, ginger, chilli & celery. Fry gently for two to three mins or until it gets softened but not coloured, then add the curry powder and cook for an additional minute.

2. Add the stock, lentils, tomatoes and simmer gently for ten mins. Well, depending on how crunchy you

want your celery you may increase or decrease the cooking time.

3. In the meantime, mix the oil, lemon juice and turmeric and then rub all over the salmon. Carefully place on a clean baking tray and then cook for eight to ten mins.

4. Stir the parsley through the celery and then serve with the salmon.

Coronation Chicken Salad

Yields: 1 Serving Overall Time: 7 Mins

Recipes:

- One teaspoon of Coriander (chopped)

- One Bird's eye chili

- One teaspoon of ground turmeric

- ¼- lemon juiceHalf teaspoon Mild curry powder

- Six Walnut halves (finely chopped)

- 75grams of Natural yoghurt

- 100grams Cooked chicken breast (cut into bite-sized pieces)

- 20grams of Red onion, diced

- 40grams of Rocket (serving purpose)

- 1 Medjool date (finely chopped)

Directions

1. Mix the coriander, lemon juice, spices and yoghurt together in a container. Add all the other recipes and serve on a bed of the rocket.

Baked Potatoes With Spicy Chickpea Stew

Yields; 4 – 6 Servings Overall Time: 1 hr

Recipes:

- Two tablespoons of olive oil

- Four to Six baking potatoes (pricked all over)

- Four cloves garlic (grated or crushed)

- Two red onions (finely chopped)

- 2-cm ginger (grated)

- Two tablespoons of cumin seeds

- Two teaspoons of chilli flakes (or as desired)

- Splash of water

- Two tablespoons of turmeric

- Two tablespoons of unsweetened cocoa powder (or cacao)

- Two (400grams) tins of chopped tomatoes

- Two yellow peppers (or desired colour and chop into bite-size pieces)

- Side salad (if desired)

- Two tablespoons parsley plus extra for garnish

- Two (400grams) tins chickpeas (or kidney beans if preferred) as well as the chickpea water (keep water)

- Salt and pepper to taste (if desired)

Directions

1. Firstly you should heat up the oven to 200 degrees Celsius, in the meantime, set all the recipes.

2. As soon as the oven is hot, Place the baking potatoes, cook for one hour or when it's cooked is you desire.

3. When the baking potatoes are in the oven, put the chopped red onion and the olive oil in a large clean

saucepan and gently cook, with the lid on for five minutes, until the onions are soften but aren't brown.

4. Take away the lid and add the ginger, garlic, chilli and cumin. On a low heat, cook for an additional minute, then add a small splash of water and the turmeric and for an additional minute, cook (Ensure the pan doesn't get dried).

5. Then, add in the cocoa powder, tomatoes, yellow pepper and chickpeas (together with the chickpea water). Bring to the boil, then proceed to simmer on a low heat for forty-five minutes until the sauce becomes thick and also unctuous (ensure it doesn't get burnt). The stew should be ready at approximately same time as the potatoes.

6. Lastly stir in the two tablespoons of parsley, pepper and some salt (if desired), and top on the baked potatoes, maybe plus a side salad.

Grape And Melon Juice

Yields: 1 Servings Overall Time: 2 minutes

Recipes:

- Half cucumber (seeds removed, roughly chopped peeled if desired)

- 30grams of young spinach leaves (stalks removed)

- 100grams of red seedless grapes

- 100grams of cantaloupe melon (peeled, deseeded & cut into chunks)

Directions

1. Blend all recipes in a blender or juicer till smoothens.

Kale And Red Onion Dhal With Buckwheat

Yields: 4 Servings Overall Time: 30 mins

Recipes:

- One small red onion (sliced)

- One tablespoon of olive oil

- Three garlic cloves (either grated or crushed)

- One bird's eye chilli (deseeded and finely chopped) if desired

- 2-cm ginger (grated)

- Two teaspoons of turmeric

- 160grams of buckwheat (or brown rice)

- 160grams of red lentils

- Two teaspoons of garam masala

- 400ml of coconut milk

- 100grams of kale (or spinach if preferred)

- 200ml of water

Directions

1. Pour the olive oil in a deep clean saucepan and add the sliced onion. Now cook on a low heat, with the lid on for five minutes until becomes softened.

2. Add the ginger, chilli and garlic and then cook for an additional minute.

3. Add the garam masala, turmeric and a little water and cook for an additional minute.

4. Add the coconut milk, 200ml water and red lentils.

5. Mix carefully all recipes and then cook for twenty minutes over a gently heat with the lid on. Occasionally stir and add you should add more water if the dhal starts to stick.

6. Kale should be added after twenty minutes, carefully stir and put the lid, cook for an additional

five minutes (one to two minutes if you use spinach as an alternative.)

7. Approximately fifteen minutes before the curry is set, place the buckwheat in a clean medium saucepan and add sufficiently of boiling water. Bring the water back to the boil, and then cook for ten minutes (you can cook longer if you enjoy your buckwheat soft). Drain the buckwheat and serve alongside the dhal.

Chargrilled Beef With A Red Wine Jus, Garlic Kale, Onion Rings, & Herb Roasted Potatoes

Recipes:

- 100grams potatoes (peeled & diced into 2-cm)

- One tablespoon of extra virgin olive oil

- 5grams of parsley (finely chopped)

- 50grams of red onion (sliced into rings)

- 50grams of kale (sliced)

- One garlic clove (finely chopped)

- 120grams beef fillet steak (3.5cm-thick)or sirloin steak (2cm-thick)

- 40ml of red wine

- 150ml of beef stock

- One teaspoon of tomato purée

- One teaspoon of cornflour, dissolved in one tablespoon of water

Directions:

1. Heat up the oven to 220 degrees Fahrenheit.

2. Carefully place the potatoes in a clean saucepan of boiling water, bring back to the boil and cook for around four to five minutes, then drain afterwards. Place in a roasting pan with one teaspoon of the oil and roast in the hot oven for thirty-five to forty-five minutes. Toss the potatoes every ten minutes to confirm even cooking. When cooked, take out from the oven, sprinkle with the chopped parsley and mix thoroughly.

3. In one teaspoon of the oil, fry the onion over medium heat for five to seven minutes, until it becomes soft and pleasantly caramelized, store warm. Steam the kale for around two to three minutes then drain. Fry the garlic lightly in half teaspoon of oil for one minute, until it becomes soft

but not coloured. Add the kale and fry for an additional one to two minutes, until it gets tender, and then, store warm.

4. You would have to heat up an ovenproof frying pan over a high heat until it begins smoke. Coat the meat in half a teaspoon of the oil and fry in the hot pan over a medium to high heat (or just as you like your meat to be). If you prefer your meat medium it is better if you sear the meat and then transfer the pan to an oven preheated at 220 degrees Fahrenheit or gas 7 and finish the cooking that way.

5. Take out the meat from the frying pan and put away to rest. Add the wine to the hot pan to bring up any meat residue. Bubble to decrease the wine by half, until syrupy & with a concentrated flavor.

6. Add tomato purée and the stock to the steak pan & bring to the boil, then add the cornflour paste to

thicken sauce, adding it a little at a time until you have your desired consistency. Carefully Stir in any of the juices from the rested steak and then serve with the roasted potatoes, kale, onion rings and also red wine sauce.

Kale And Blackcurrant Smoothie

Yields: 2 Servings Overall Time: 3 Minutes

Recipes:

- Two teaspoons of honey

- One cup of freshly made green tea

- Ten baby kale leaves (stalks removed)

- One ripe banana

- 40grams of blackcurrants (rinsed & stalks removed)

- Six ice cubes

Directions:

Gently stir in the honey into the warm green tea until it gets dissolved. Whiz all other recipes together in a clean blender until it smoothens. Serve straight away.

Buckwheat Pasta Salad

Yields: 1 Serving

Recipes:

- One large handful of rocket

- 50grams of buckwheat pasta (cooked according to the packet directions)

- Eight cherry tomatoes (halved)

- One small handful of basil leaves

- 20grams of pine nuts

- Ten olives

- Half of avocado (diced)

- One tablespoons of extra virgin olive oil

Directions:

Gently combine all the recipes excluding the pine nuts and then arrange on a dish or in a container, then sprinkle the pine nuts all over it.

Greek Salad Skewers

Yields: 2 Servings Overall Time: 10 Minutes

Recipes:

- Eight large black olives

- Two wooden skewers (soaked in water for thirty minutes before usage)

- One yellow pepper (cut into eight squares)

- 100grams of cucumber (cut into four slices & halved)

- Eight cherry tomatoes

- 100grams of feta (cut into eight cubes)

- Half red onion (cut in half & separated into eight pieces)

For The Dressing:

- Half lemon juice

- One tablespoon of extra virgin olive oil

- Half clove garlic (peeled & crushed)

- One teaspoon of balsamic vinegar

- Few leaves oregano (finely chopped)

- Freshly ground black pepper

- Enough salt for seasoning

- Few leaves basil, finely chopped (or half teaspoon of dried mixed herbs to replace basil & oregano)

Directions

1. You should firstly thread every skewer with the salad recipes in the order as follows: olive, tomato,

yellow pepper, red onion, cucumber, feta, tomato, olive, yellow pepper, red onion, cucumber, feta.

2. Lastly, place all the dressing recipes in a small clean container and mix together

3. completely. Pour over the skewers afterwards.

Kale, Edamame And Tofu Curry

Yields: 4 Servings Overall Time: 45 Minutes

Recipes:

- One large onion (chopped)

- One tablespoon of rapeseed oil

- One large thumb fresh ginger (peeled & grated)

- Four cloves garlic (peeled & grated)

- Half teaspoon of ground turmeric

- One red chilli, (deseeded & thinly sliced)

- One teaspoon of paprika

- 1/4 teaspoon of cayenne pepper

- One teaspoon of salt

- Half teaspoon of ground cumin

- 200grams of kale leaves (stalks removed & torn)

- One litre of boiling water

- 250grams of dried red lentils

- 200grams firm tofu (chopped into cubes)

- 50grams frozen soyaedamame beans

- One lime juice

- Two tomatoes (roughly chopped)

Directions

1. Firstly put the oil in a clean heavy-bottomed pan over a low to medium heat. Add the onion and cook for five minutes before adding the ginger, chilli and garlic and cooking for an additional 2 minutes. Add the, cayenne, turmeric, cumin, salt and paprika. Stir before adding the red lentils and then stirring once more.

2. Secondly, pour in the boiling water and bring to a hearty simmer for ten minutes, then decrease the heat and cook for an additional twenty to thirty

minutes until the curry gets so thick just like porridge.

3. Then lastly, add the tofu, tomatoes and soya beans and cook for an additional 5 minutes. Add the kale leaves and lime (juice) and cook until the kale gets tender.

Chocolate Cupcakes With Matcha Icing

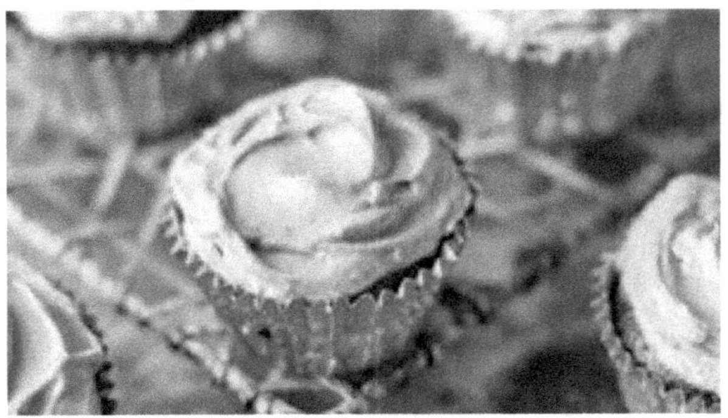

Yields: 12 Servings Overall Time: 35 Minutes

Recipes:

- 200grams of caster sugar

- 150grams of self-raising flour

- Half teaspoon of salt

- 60grams of cocoa

- 120ml of milk

- Half teaspoon of fine espresso coffee (decaf if preferred)

- 50ml of vegetable oil

- Half teaspoon of vanilla extract

- 120ml of boiling water

- One egg

For the icing:

- 50grams of icing sugar

- 50grams of butter

- 50grams of soft cream cheese

- Half teaspoon of vanilla bean paste

- One tablespoon of matcha green tea powder

Directions

1. Firstly you will have to heat up the oven to 180 degrees Celsius. Gently line a cupcake tin with clean paper or silicone cake cases.

2. Place the sugar, flour, salt, espresso powder and cocoa in a large clean container and mix vigorously.

3. Add the vanilla extract, milk, egg and vegetable oil to the dry recipes and use a clean electric mixer to beat until combined well. Gently pour in the boiling water gradually and beat on a low speed until it is thoroughly combined. At high speed to beat for an additional minute to add air to the batter (batter is much more liquid than a regular cake mix).

4. Spoon the batter equally between the cake cases. Every cake case should be no more than ¾ full.

Bake in the oven for fifteen to eighteen minutes, until the mixture bounces back when tapped. Take out from the oven and then allow it cool totally before icing.

5. For the icing, cream icing sugar and the butter together until it appears pale and gets smoothen. Add the vanilla and matcha powder and stir once more. Lastly add the cream cheese and then beat until it smoothens. Spread or pipe over the cakes.

Sesame Chicken Salad

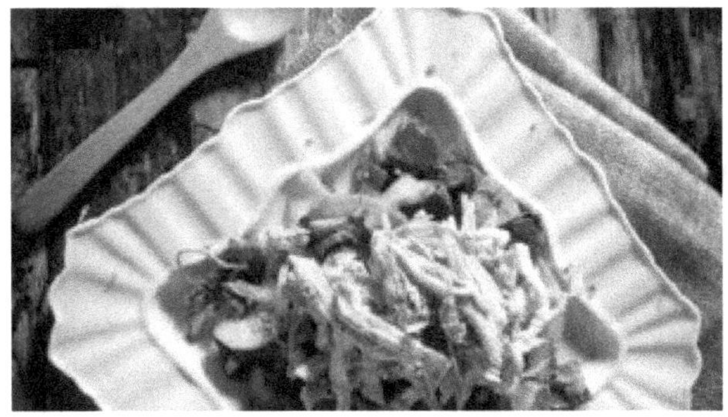

Yields: 2 Servings Overall Time: 12 Minutes

Recipes:

- One cucumber (peeled, halved, deseeded and sliced)

- One tablespoon of sesame seeds

- 60grams pak choi, (very finely shredded)

- 100grams baby kale (roughly chopped)

- Half red onion (very finely sliced)

- 150grams of cooked chicken, shredded

- Large handful parsley (chopped)

For the dressing:

- One teaspoon of sesame oil

- One tablespoon of extra virgin olive oil

- One lime juice

- Two teaspoons of soy sauce

- One teaspoon of clear honey

Directions

1. Firstly you will have to toast the sesame seeds in a dry clean frying pan for two minutes until it appears lightly browned and begins to fragrant. Transfer to a dish to cool.

2. In a clean small container, mix together the sesame oil, olive oil, honey, soy sauce and lime juice to make the dressing.

3. Place the kale, cucumber, red onion, parsley and pak choi in a clean large container and gradually mix together. Afterward pour over the dressing and mix once again.

4. Share the salad between 2 plates and also top with the shredded chicken. Sprinkling over the sesame seeds before serving.

SirtFood Mushroom Scramble Eggs

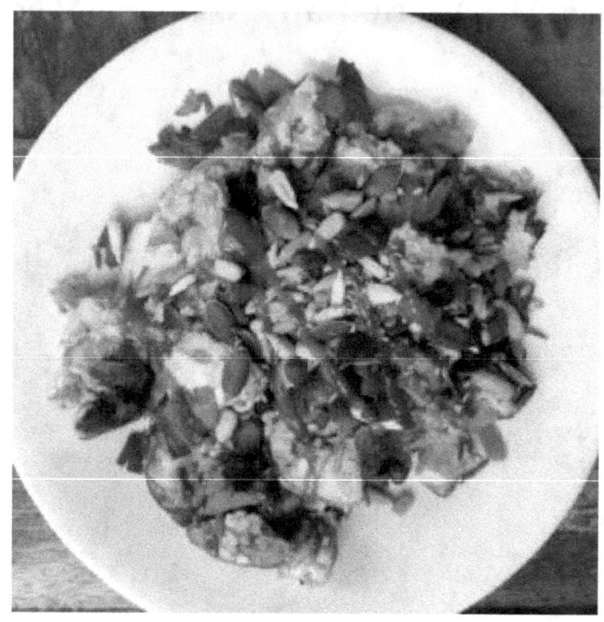

Recipes:

- One teaspoon of ground turmeric

- Two eggs

- 20grams of kale (roughly chopped)

- One teaspoon of mild curry powder

- Half of bird's eye chilli (thinly sliced)

- One teaspoon of extra virgin olive oil

- 5grams of parsley (finely chopped)

- Handful of button mushrooms (thinly sliced)

- A seed mixture as a topper & some Rooster Sauce for flavor (if desired)

Directions

1. Firstly you should mix the curry powder and turmeric and add water until you have attained a light paste.

2. Secondly, steam the kale for two to three minutes.

3. Lastly, Heat the oil in a clean frying pan over a medium heat and fry the mushrooms and chilli for two to three minutes until it begins to appear brown and gets soften.

Aromatic Chicken Breast with Kale, Red Onion & Salsa

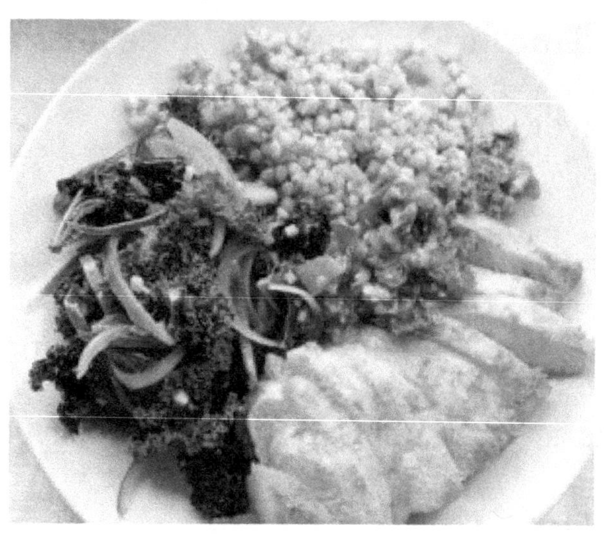

Recipes:

- Two teaspoons of ground turmeric

- 120grams of skinless (boneless chicken breast)

- One tablespoon of extra virgin olive oil

- ¼ of lemon juice

- 50grams of buckwheat

- 20grams of red onion (sliced)

- 50grams of kale (chopped)

- One teaspoon of chopped fresh ginger

Directions:

To make the salsa:

1. Firstly, remove the eye from the tomato and then chop it very finely, keep as much of the liquid as possible. Mix with the capers, chilli, lemon juice and parsley. You could put all in a clean blender but the end outcome is a little changed.

2. Secondly, you should heat up the oven to 220 degrees Celsius. Marinate the chicken breast in one teaspoon of the turmeric, the lemon juice and a little oil. Leave for five to ten minutes.

3. Thirdly, heat a clean ovenproof frying pan until it gets hot, then add the marinated chicken and cook for one minute or thereabout on each side, until it appears pale golden, afterwards transfer to the oven (place on a clean baking tray if not an ovenproof pan) for eight to ten minutes, until it is well cooked. Take it out from the oven, then cover with foil and let it rest for five minutes before serving.

4. Cook the kale in a steamer for five minutes. Fry the ginger and red onions in oil, until it becomes soft but isn't coloured, afterwards add the cooked kale and then fry for further minute.

5. Cook the buckwheat according to the packet directions with the left teaspoon of turmeric. Serve together with the vegetables, salsa and chicken.

Smoked Salmon Omelette

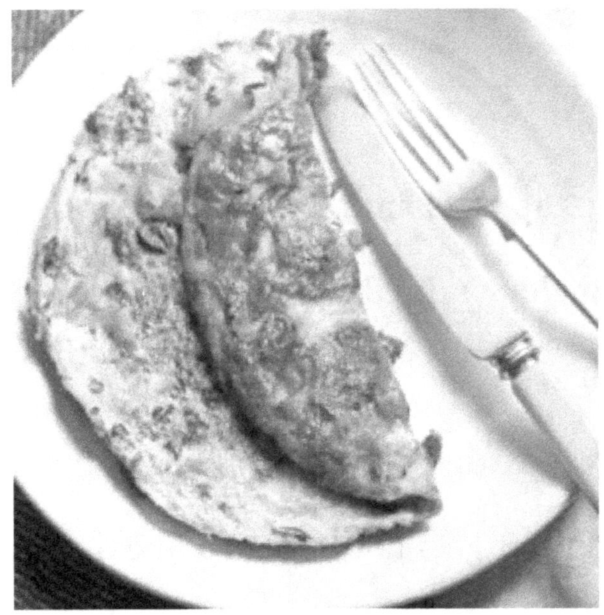

Yields: 1 Serving Overall Time: 5 to 10 Minutes

Recipes:

- 100grams of smoked salmon (sliced)

- Two Medium eggs

- 10grams of Rocket (chopped)

- Half teaspoon of Capers

- One teaspoon of Extra virgin olive oil

- One teaspoon of Parsley (chopped)

Directions

1. Crack the eggs into a clean container and whisk thoroughly. Add the capers, salmon, parsley and rocket.

2. Lastly, heat the olive oil in a clean non-stick frying pan until it gets hot but isn't smoking. Add the egg mixture and using fish slice or a spatula, move the mixture around the pan until it is even. Decrease the heat and let the omelette cook well. Slide the spatula about the edges and fold or roll up the omelette in half to serve.

Green Tea Smoothie

Yields: 2 Servings Overall Time: 3 Minutes

Recipes:

- Two ripe bananas

- 250ml of milk

- Six ice cubes

- Two teaspoons of matcha green tea powder

- Two teaspoons of honey

- Half teaspoon of vanilla bean paste (not extract) or a small scrape of the seeds from a vanilla pod

Directions:

Just blend all the recipes together in a clean blender and serve in 2 clean glasses.

Eating Plan

The Sirtfood diet is designed for a period of three weeks, but the nutritional principles can be used to sustain maintenance for a long time. How do you begin the diet of Sirtfood?

First Phase (Days 1–3):

- ❖ Calorie consumption reduced in the first three days of the diet to 1,000 calories a day

- ❖ Take three cups of green juice Sirtfood a day

- ❖ Consuming one rich Sirtfood meal a day

- ❖ 15grams to 20grams of dark chocolate is allowed (85% cocoa).

First Phase (Days 4–7):

* Limit calorie intake to 1,500 calories a day (500 more calories than during the first three days) on days 4–7

* Drink two sirtfood green juices per day

* Eat two sirtfood-rich meals per day

* 15grams to 20grams of dark chocolate is allowed (85% cocoa).

Second Phase (Lasts Two Weeks):

* Once you complete the first week, there is no strict long-term schedule. You are advised to eat three nutritious foods and continue to drink sirtfood.

* It is advised that you continue to use plenty of sirtfood in your diet, though you stick to more balanced, herbal foods.

* In fact, this diet will proceed forever as long as you consume enough calories to satisfy your needs.

7 Days Meal Plan

So how does it work?

For the first three days, calorie consumption is reduced to 1.000 calories per day, including three sirt foods green juices plus sirtfood and antioxidant-packed sirtfood snacks.

For the last 4 days, you raise your calorie consumption to 1500 calories a day by eating two sirtfood meals and two green juices, thereby cutting off the bites.

The future

You can carry out this plan for up to two weeks and then adjust it according to your lifestyle.

No rules – just try to include as many sirtfoods as possible in your diet, making your skin healthier, more energetic, more lean and better.

Clients who continued with the diet experienced continuous and sustained weight loss over 2nd stage.

This super healthy green juice and these delicious bites are the staples of Sirtfood Diet.

All recipes serve one (unless otherwise stated).

Sirtfood Green Juice

Recipes:

- 30grams of rocket

- 75grams of kale

- Half medium green apple

- 5grams of flat-leaf parsley

- 5grams of lovage leaves (if desired)

- Half teaspoon of matcha green tea

- 150grams celery including leaves

- Half lemon juice

Directions

1. Juice the rocket, kale, lovage and parsley, if using, then add the apple and celery and blend once more. You should squeeze in the lemon in the blend.

2. Pour a little amount of the juice into a clean glass, then add the matcha into the glass and then stir

until it gets dissolved. Add the left juice and serve straightaway.

Note

In the first two drinks of the day-use just matcha, as it contains the same caffeine content as a regular cup of tea. If you don't get used to it, it can keep you awake later in the day if you get drunk.

Yields: (makes 15-20 bites)

Recipes:

- 30grams of dark chocolate (85percent of cocoa solids), broken into pieces, or cocoa nibs

- 120grams of walnuts

- One tablespoon of cocoa powder

- 250grams of Medjool dates (pitted)

- One tablespoon of extra virgin olive oil

- Scraped seeds of one vanilla pod or 1tsp vanilla extract

- One tablespoon of ground turmeric

Directions:

1. Place the chocolate and walnuts into a clean food processor and blend until you achieve a fine powder. Add all the other recipes and blend until the mixture makes a big ball. Add two tablespoons of water to help bind it, if required.

2. Make bite-sized balls with your hands from mixture and cool them in an airtight jar for at least one hour before serving. The balls are stored in the fridge for up to a week.

Day 1

Sirtfood green juices – 3 Times

Sirtfood bites – 2 Times (you can replace these for 15grams to 20grams of dark chocolate if you desired)

Sirtfood meal – 1 Times

Asian King Prawn Stir-Fry

Recipes:

- Two teaspoons of tamari or soy sauce

- 150grams of raw king prawns (shelled)

- One clove garlic (finely chopped)

- Two teaspoons of extra virgin olive oil

- One tsp fresh ginger (finely chopped)

- One bird's eye chili (finely chopped)

- 40grams of celery (trimmed and sliced)

- 5grams of lovage or celery leaves

- 20grams of red onion (sliced)

- 75grams of green beans (chopped)

- 75grams of soba (buckwheat noodles)

- 100ml of chicken stock

- 50grams of kale, roughly chopped

Directions

1. In a large clean frying pan over high heat, carefully cook the prawns in one teaspoon of tamari or soy sauce and one teaspoon of oil for two to three minutes. Transfer to a clean dish.

2. Add the left oil to the pan and fry the chili, garlic, red onion, ginger, celery, kale and beans over medium to high heat for two to three minutes. Add the stock & bring to the boil, then simmer until the vegetables are cooked but remains crunchy.

3. In boiling water, cook the noodles following the packet directions. Drain and add the celery leaves or lovage, prawns and noodles to the pan. Bring back to the boil, then take away from the heat and serve it.

Day 2

Sirtfood green juices – 3 Times

Sirtfood bites – 2 Times

Sirtfood meal – 1 Time

Turkey Escalope

Recipes:

- 150grams of cauliflower (roughly chopped)

- One clove garlic (finely chopped)

- 40grams of red onion (finely chopped)

- One bird's eye chili (finely chopped)

- One teaspoon of fresh ginger (finely chopped)

- Two tablespoons of extra virgin olive oil

- Two teaspoons of ground turmeric

- 30grams of sun-dried tomatoes (finely chopped)

- 10grams of parsley

- 150grams of turkey escalope

- One teaspoon of dried sage

- Half lemon juice

- One tablespoon of capers

Directions

1. In a clean food processor place the cauliflower and pulse in 2-second bursts to finely chop it until it looks like couscous. Put aside. Fry the red onion, chili, ginger and garlic in one teaspoon of the oil until becomes soft but isn't coloured. Add the cauliflower and turmeric and cook for one minute. Remove from the heat and then add the sun-dried tomatoes and half the parsley.

2. Coat the turkey escalope in the left oil and sage then fry for five to six minutes, consistently turning. After it is cooked, add the remaining parsley, lemon juice,

one tablespoon of water and capers to the pan to

prepare a sauce, and then serve.

Sirtfood green juices – 3 Times

Sirtfood bites – 2 Times

Sirtfood meal – 1 Time

Aromatic Chicken

Recipes:

For the salsa:

- One bird's eye chili (finely chopped)

- One large tomato

- One tablespoon of capers (finely chopped)

- Half lemon juice

- 5grams of parsley (finely chopped)

For the chicken:

- Two teaspoons of ground turmeric

- 120grams of skinless, boneless chicken breast

- One tablespoon of extra virgin olive oil

- Half lemon juice

- 20grams of red onion (sliced)

- 50grams of buckwheat

- 50grams of kale (chopped)

- One teaspoon of fresh ginger (finely chopped)

Directions

1. Firstly you should heat up the oven to 220 degrees Fahrenheit.

2. For the salsa, chop the tomato finely, keep enough liquid. Mix with the capers, chili, lemon juice and parsley.

3. The chicken breast should be marinated in one teaspoon of the turmeric, lemon juice and half the oil for five to ten minutes.

4. Afterward, heat up a clean ovenproof frying pan, add the marinated chicken and cook for one minute on every side until it appears golden, then move to the oven for eight to ten minutes or until it is well cooked. Take out from the oven, cover with foil and let it rest for five minutes.

5. Cook the kale in a steamer for five minutes. Fry the ginger and onion in the rest of the oil until gets soft but isn't coloured, then add the cooked kale and then fry for an additional minute.

6. Following the pack directions cook the buckwheat with the remaining turmeric, and serve when ready.

Day 4

Sirtfood green juices – 3 Times

Sirtfood meal – 2 Times

Sirt Muesli

Recipes:

- 10grams of buckwheat puffs

- 20grams of buckwheat flakes

- 40grams of Medjool dates (pitted and chopped)

- 15grams of coconut flakes or desiccated coconut

- 100grams of plain Greek yogurt (for vegan: soya or coconut yogurt)

- 15grams of walnuts (chopped)

- 100grams of strawberries (hulled and chopped)

- 10grams of cocoa nibs

Directions

Mix all of the recipes together and serve immediately.

Note:

Leave out the yogurt and strawberries if you aren't serving immediately.

Pan-fried Salmon Salad

Recipes:

For the dressing:

- Half lemon juice

- 10grams of parsley

- One tablespoon of extra virgin olive oil

- One tablespoon of capers

For the salad:

- 100grams of cherry tomatoes (halved)

- Half avocado (peeled, stoned and diced)

- 50grams of rocket

- 20grams of red onion (thinly sliced)

- 150grams of skinless salmon fillet

- 70grams of chicory (head), halved

- 5grams of celery leaves

- Two teaspoons of brown sugar

Directions

1. Firstly, you should heat the oven to 220 degrees Fahrenheit.

2. For the dressing, whizz the capers, lemon juice, parsley and two teaspoons of oil in a clean blender until it is smooth.

3. For the salad, mix the tomato, avocado, rocket, celery leaves and red onion together.

4. Coat the salmon with small oil and sear it in a clean ovenproof frying pan for one minute. Move to a clean baking tray and then cook in the oven for five minutes.

5. Mix the brown sugar with one teaspoon of oil & brush it over the cut sides of the chicory. Gently place the cut-sides down in a hot frying pan & then cook for two to three minutes, frequently turning. Dress the salad & serve together.

Day 5

Sirtfood green juices – 3 Times

Sirtfood meal – 2 Times

Strawberry Tabbouleh

Recipes:

- One tablespoon of ground turmeric

- 50grams of buckwheat

- 65grams of tomato

- 80grams of avocado

- 100grams of strawberries, hulled

- 20grams of red onion

- One tablespoon of capers

- One tablespoon of extra virgin olive oil

- 25grams of Medjool dates, pitted

- 30grams of rocket

- 30grams of parsley

- Half lemon juice

Directions:

1. Firstly, you should cook the buckwheat with the turmeric following the pack directions. Drain and let it cool.

2. Finely chop the tomato, avocado, dates, red onion, parsley and capers and then mix with the buckwheat.

3. Lastly, slice the strawberries and slowly mix into the salad with the lemon juice and oil. Serve on the rocket.

Miso-marinated Baked Cod

Recipes:

- One tablespoon of mirin

- 20grams of miso

- 200grams of skinless cod fillet

- One tablespoon of extra virgin olive oil

- 40grams of celery (sliced)

- 20grams of red onion (sliced)

- One bird's eye chili (finely chopped)

- One clove garlic (finely chopped)

- One tablespoon of tamari or soy sauce

- One teaspoon of fresh ginger (finely chopped)

- 50grams of kale (roughly chopped)

- One teaspoon of sesame seeds

- 30grams of buckwheat

- One teaspoon of ground turmeric

- 60grams of green beans

- 5grams of parsley (roughly chopped)

Directions:

1. Firstly, you should heat up the oven to 220 degrees Celsius.

2. Mix the mirin, miso and one teaspoon of oil, rub into the cod and marinate for thirty minutes. Move to a clean baking tray and then cook for ten minutes.

3. Afterward, heat up a clean large frying pan with the oil left. Add the onion and stir-fry for some minutes, then add the garlic, celery, ginger, chili, kale and green beans. Fry until the kale gets tender and is

well cooked, adding some water to soften the kale if required.

4. Cook the buckwheat following to pack directions with the turmeric. Add the parsley, tamari or soy sauce and sesame seeds to the stir-fry and serve with the fish and greens.

Day 6

Sirtfood green juices – 3 Times

Sirtfood meal – 2 Times

Sirt Super Salad

Recipes:

- 50grams of chicory leaves

- 50grams of rocket

- 80grams of avocado (peeled, stoned and sliced)

- 100grams of smoked salmon slices

- 20grams of red onion (sliced)

- 40grams of celery (sliced)

- One tablespoon of capers

- 10grams of lovage or celery leaves (chopped)

- 15grams of walnuts (chopped)

- 10grams of parsley (chopped)

- One tablespoon of extra virgin olive oil

- One large Medjool date (pitted and chopped)

- Half lemon juice

Direction

Mix all the recipes together and then serve.

Recipes:

- One tablespoon of extra virgin olive oil

- 100grams of potatoes (peeled and diced)

- 50grams of red onion (sliced into rings)

- 5grams of parsley (finely chopped)

- One clove garlic (finely chopped)

- 50grams of kale (chopped)

- Steak or 2 cm-thick sirloin steaks

- One teaspoon of cornflour, dissolved in one teaspoon of water

- 40ml of red wine

- 120grams -150grams beef fillet

- 150ml of beef stock

- One teaspoon of tomato purée

Directions

1. Firstly, you should heat up the oven to 220 degrees Celsius.

2. Place the potatoes in a clean saucepan of boiling water, bring to the boil and cook for four to five minutes, then drain. Place in a clean roasting tin with one teaspoon of oil and cook for thirty-five to forty-five minutes, turning every 10 minutes. Take out from the oven, sprinkle with the chopped parsley and mix gently.

3. Fry the onion in one teaspoon of oil over medium heat until gets soft and caramelised. Keep warm.

4. Steam the kale for around two to three minutes, then drain. Fry the garlic gently in half teaspoon of

oil for one minute until gets soft. Add the kale and fry for an additional one to two minutes, until becomes tender. Store warm.

5. Now heat a clean ovenproof frying pan until it begins to smoke. Coat the meat in half teaspoon of oil and fry depending how you prefer your meat done. Take out from the pan and put aside. Add the wine to the hot pan bring up any meat remainder. Bubble to decrease the wine by half until it's syrupy with a concentrated flavour.

6. Add tomato purée and the stock to the steak pan and also bring to the boil, then gently add the cornflour paste to thicken the sauce a little at a time until you have the preferred consistency. Carefully stir in any juice from the rested steak and serve with the kale, potatoes, red wine sauce and onion rings.

Day 7

Sirtfood green juices – 3 Times

Sirtfood meal – 2 Times

Sirtfood Omelet

Recipes:

- Three medium eggs

- 50grams of streaky bacon

- One teaspoon of extra virgin olive oil

- 5grams of parsley (finely chopped)

- 35grams of red chicory (thinly sliced)

Directions

1. Heat a clean non-stick frying pan. Carefully cut the bacon into thin strips & then cook over high heat until crispy. No need to add any oil – there should be enough fat in the bacon to cook it. Take out from the pan and place on a clean kitchen paper to drain any excess fat. Wipe the pan clean.

2. Gently whisk the eggs and mix with the parsley and chicory. Carefully stir the cooked bacon through the eggs.

3. In a large clean non-stick frying pan, heat the oil, and then add the egg mixture. Cook until the omelet becomes firm.

4. Ease the spatula around the edges and then fold the omelet in half or roll up and serve to enjoy.

Baked Chicken Breast

Recipes:

For The Pesto:

- 15grams of walnuts

- 15grams of parsley

- 15grams of Parmesan

- One tablespoon of extra virgin olive oil

- Half lemon juice

For The Chicken:

- 20grams of red onions, finely sliced

- 150grams of skinless chicken breast

- 35grams of rocket

- One teaspoon of red wine vinegar

- One teaspoon of balsamic vinegar

- 100grams of cherry tomatoes, halved

Directions

1. Firstly you should heat up the oven to 220 degrees Celsius.

To Make The Pesto:

2. Blend the walnuts, parsley, olive oil, Parmesan, one tablespoon of water and half the lemon juice in a clean food processor until a smooth paste is achieved. You can add more water if required.

3. Now, you should marinate the chicken breast in one tablespoon of the pesto and the lemon juice in the refrigerator for thirty minutes or more.

4. Fry the chicken in its marinade in a clean ovenproof frying pan over medium to high heat, for one minute on each side, afterwards, move the pan to the oven and then cook for eight minutes, or just until it is well cooked.

5. In the red wine vinegar, marinate the onions for five to ten minutes, ensure you drain off the liquid afterwards.

6. As soon as the chicken is well cooked, take out from the oven, spoon over one tablespoon of pesto, allowing the pesto to be melted by the heat from the chicken. Gently cover with a clean foil and then leave to rest for five minutes before serving it.

7. Combine the tomatoes, onion and rocket and then drizzle over the balsamic. Serve alongside the chicken, spooning over the rest of the pesto.

21 Days Meal Plan

Want to keep going?

Over the next 14 days, ensure you take;

- One green juice

- Three sirtfood meals per day.

Conclusion

This Sirtfood Diet CookBook would serve as a guide to weight loss and will give you amazing ideas for delicious recipes

The recipes are adequate for all cooking skill levels and are great to prepare with the families.

Get lean and stay healthy.

Enjoy!

www.ingramcontent.com/pod-product-compliance
Lightning Source LLC
Chambersburg PA
CBHW070843250726
48662CB00003B/1337